Fatty Liver Diet:

Guide on How to End Fatty Liver Disease

Table of Contents

Additionally, the information in the following pages is intended only for informational purposes and should thus be thought of as universal. As befitting its nature, it is presented without assurance regarding its prolonged validity or interim quality. Trademarks that are mentioned are done without written consent and in no way be considered an endorsement from the trademark holder.

BONUS:

As a way of saying thank you for purchasing my book, please use your link below to claim your 3 FREE Cookbooks on Health, Fitness & Dieting Instantly

https://bit.ly/2LEQVu2

You can also share your link with your friends and families whom you think that can benefit from the cookbooks or you can forward them the link as a gift!

Introduction

Taking an active role in your health is important. If you are worried about your liver, you may have heard about doing a liver detox, cleanse or flush. Your liver, the second largest organ in your body, processes external medicine and internal nutrients in addition to making sure your body removes potentially harmful toxins. Many people decide to do a liver detox after extended consumption of processed foods alcohol in order to assist their body in removing these toxins. Other people turn to a liver detox to assist their daily life. Additionally, others consider a liver detox when they have developed a liver disease and are looking for additional treatment options.

Similar to other detoxes, there are variations available and certain things you need to know before beginning. For example, there are different foods and drinks that are good for supporting your liver's health, and other foods and drinks that can be harmful. Some detoxes are best for a single day while others can last up to a week or more. Some are actually very unhealthy for your body while others support your nutritional needs. These are just some of the reasons why you need to pay attention to what you choose to do to detox your liver and also support your overall health.

Detoxing your liver helps you in a variety of ways. First, you will most likely begin to feel better early in the process. You will feel lighter, healthier, and energetic. Second, you will help your body begin to adjust to a healthy diet instead of existing on unhealthy foods and drinks. Finally, you will begin to remove excess toxins and fat build up from your body.

The reason you experience these amazing benefits is that a liver detox, especially ones focused on your over health and liver function, removes processed foods and alcohol from your diet for a period of time. Foods and drinks in these categories are high-calorie, high-sugar, and high-fat foods that do not deliver a proportional level of nutrients. Other benefits include a focus on whole foods which means many foods people are sensitive to are removed. For example, most detoxes require you to cease eating gluten-rich foods and dairy.

Your liver is critically important to the function of your body, and doing a liver detox is a great natural way to support healthy liver function and heal damage to your liver. It is not always possible to repair existing damage, but detoxes can prevent future damage and support your general health in the meantime.

Doctors say liver detoxes aren't important for your health or how well your liver works. There's no proof they help get rid of toxins after you've had too much food or alcohol. There's also no evidence that they fix the liver damage that has already happened.

A Few Things to Know About the Safety of Liver Detoxes

If you already have a liver disease, you are should be working closely with your medical team to treat your liver. Talk with them about a liver cleanse and make sure to remain under their supervision while completing the detox. Make sure you choose a detox that is good for you with a focus on nutrition and health instead of weight loss or chemical additives. Other considerations include:

- Beware of liver-detox products available for sale in a store. These can contain harmful ingredients and also may make false claims regarding the safety and effectiveness of the product.
- A juice that is unpasteurized has the potential to make you ill. The risk increases for people who have a weak immune system and also for the elderly.
- Other illnesses can be made worse by a liver detox. For example, a 24-hour liver detox juice cleanse can irritate and worsen a pre-existing kidney disease. Fasting before or during the detox can worsen hepatitis B. If you have any other illnesses and are considering doing a liver detox, make sure to talk with your medical professional about any potential conflicts with doing the detox.
- Diabetes is another disease that requires medical intervention and supervision. Again, make sure you work with your medical team to make sure your detox does not interfere with any other medical condition, like diabetes.
- Side effects including dehydration, headaches, light-headed, or weakness, can occur, especially if you choose to fast as part of the process.

Keep Your Liver Healthy

Your liver's health is determined by your genetics and general health. Your environment, lifestyle, and diet also affect your liver's health. There are things you can do before, during and after your detox to help support your overall health and your liver health. Some of the following guidelines are beneficial, especially if you are predisposed to the liver disease. For example, a history of liver disease in your family or excessive alcohol consumption can make it more likely that you develop the fatty liver disease. The guidelines are as follows:

1. Cut back on your alcohol consumption.
2. Every day, focus on eating a diet that is well balanced. This includes protein, whole grains, seeds, nuts, fresh vegetables, and fruits.
3. Obtain and maintain a healthy weight for your age, gender, and height.
4. Try to get moderate to high levels of exercise every day. If you have been inactive or only minimally active, make sure to work with your medical professional before adopting any new lifestyle change.
5. Hepatitis is very dangerous to your general health but especially harmful to your liver. Minimize the likelihood of contracting hepatitis by:
    a. Avoid unprotected sex with people you do not know well.
    b. Patronize reputable and sterile tattoo parlors for any tattoo you get.
    c. Use your own personal household items, toothbrushes, and razors.
    d. Do not use illegal drugs. If you decide to utilize them, do not share straws or needles with others.

The Main Reasons for Completing a Liver Detox for Preventing and Curing Fatty Liver Disease

1. **Lose weight.**

    Bile is what removes fat and toxins from your body and your liver produces bile. This means, in order to lose weight, you need to produce enough bile to get it out of your body. If you have been struggling with losing weight, this could be the reason.

2. **Remove liver stones.**

   Your lover does not just build up fat; it can also build up cholesterol. This creates liver stones and that can be incredibly painful and detrimental to your health.

3. **Overall body detox and health support.**

   When you do a detox, you remove toxins from your body. Any excess toxins can harm your body in multiple places. This is why a liver detox promotes your health in all areas.

4. **Improves energy levels.**

5. **The liver moves toxins out and nutrients through your body.**

   When it does not function properly due to fat buildup, nutrients may not be making it into your bloodstream as you need. This can make you feel sluggish and fatigued. When you get your liver functioning again, it is likely the increase in nutrients reaching your body will also boost your energy levels.

6. **Makes your appear and feel younger.**

   Your liver affects the health and appearance of your skin. When your liver is healthy, your skin looks and feels healthier. This external improvement helps you look and feel younger.

Chapter 1: What Is Fatty Liver Disease?

Simply defined, the fatty liver disease is a liver condition caused by a fat buildup in the organ. The human body has only one other organ that is larger than the liver, skin, and no internal organs larger than the liver. The many functions of the liver include disposing of harmful toxins, processing fat from the bloodstream and helping in the blood clotting function.

When the liver stops working correctly, fat begins to build up. Some of the reasons the liver stops working correctly include alcohol, hepatitis C, reactions to various medications, and rare metabolic issues. Conditions during pregnancy can also cause fat build up in the liver for women. There is a special category designated for other situations that lead to fat build up in the liver; NAFLD or Non-Alcoholic Fatty Liver Disease. Fat is usually built up in the liver due to obesity, diabetes, or pre-diabetes. Because of America's rise in metabolic syndromes and obesity, many doctors believe these are why the fatty liver disease is also on the rise.

Alcohol-Related Fatty Liver Disease or ALD

ALD, or alcohol-related fatty liver disease, is caused by the heavy consumption of alcohol over time. ALD symptoms include pain in the liver and belly or an enlarged liver. The symptoms and effects of the alcohol-related fatty liver disease will usually get better over time if the person discontinues drinking alcohol. If that person keeps drinking, ALD can lead to alcoholic hepatitis or alcoholic cirrhosis. Alcoholic cirrhosis of the liver can ultimately lead to liver failure, which can lead to death. ALD can comprise of alcoholic cirrhosis, acute alcoholic hepatitis, and simple hepatic steatosis. Having all these illnesses at once is feasible.

When someone abstains from alcohol, the liver will usually go back to regular. Despite the excellent prognosis for alcohol steatosis in the short-term, when patients were followed after treatment, it was found that those with changes to their lives because of alcohol abuse in the past were more likely to develop cirrhosis than others with normal liver function. Doctors use continued alcohol abuse, gender, and extreme steatosis to predict the risk factors of the patient to develop cirrhosis and fibrosis. Females have a higher risk than males.

When the liver has been severely damaged for an extended period of time, most medical professionals considered the outcome of alcoholic cirrhosis is irreversible. Studies are now being conducted that indicate some outcomes, such as cirrhosis and fibrosis, can be reversed depending on the cause and the patient. For example, the patients studied with decompensated alcoholic cirrhosis who got a liver transplant experienced outcomes similar to other liver transplant patients. Their five-year survival rate was about 70%.

The manifest symptoms of alcoholic hepatitis vary because of the disease's wide range in severity. Vomit, nausea, abdomen distention and pain, weight loss, and anorexia are mild, nonspecific symptoms. Encephalopathy, fever, spider angioma, ascites, jaundice, hepatic failure, and hepatology are more specific and severe symptoms. Encephalopathy, fever, spider angioma, ascites, jaundice, and hepatomegaly are noticeable physical symptoms.

Alcoholic hepatitis or fatty liver disease does not always precede established alcoholic cirrhosis. It can begin decompensation without the presence of either. Additionally, acute alcoholic hepatitis may be diagnosed with alcoholic cirrhosis. Other causes of cirrhosis cannot be differentiated from the signs and symptoms of alcoholic cirrhosis. Some of the symptoms and signs of patients include:

- Portal hypertension complications; for example, hepatic encephalopathy, ascites, and variceal bleeding.
- Unusual lab results; for example, coagulopathy, hypoalbuminemia, and thrombocytopenia.
- Pruritus
- Jaundice

A patient who is being evaluated for unusual liver functions test results, such as elevated aminotransferase levels, is the most common diagnostic method for fatty liver disease. There is no specific test available for the fatty liver disease. Most often it is diagnosed when a patient's aminotransferase levels are more than double the normal limits and the results from an ultrasonography. Typically, the findings of an ultrasonography reveal a liver with hyperechoic and may or may not have hepatomegaly.

MRIs or magnetic resonance imaging, and CT scans or computed technology scans are used to diagnose cirrhosis. When reviewing the results of the MRI, unique characteristics can potentially be present with alcohol-related liver disease. For example, it is noticeable if a patient's liver has a larger caudate lobe, the hepatic notch on the right side is more obvious, or the regenerative nodules are larger. It is not typically necessary to conduct a liver biopsy to diagnose fatty liver disease; however, it may be requested to determine fibrosis or steatohepatitis is not present.

Necrosis and inflammation of the liver are the most common and recognizable symptoms of alcoholic hepatitis. These features are the most noticeable in the hepatic acinus' centrilobular region. Reversible portal hypertension and sinusoid compression occur when the hepatocytes become typically distended. Inflammatory cells permeate mononuclear cells and polymorphonuclear cells. These inflammatory cells are typically situated near the necrotic hepatocytes and in the sinusoids. Mallory bodies and fatty infiltration are also often present in patients with alcoholic hepatitis. Mallory bodies are aggregations of the intracellular perinuclear, which is hematoxylin-eosin staining by eosinophilic intermediate filaments. These results are additional indicators of alcoholic hepatitis, but are not required to diagnose the disease nor are particular to the illness.

For patients that abuse alcohol significantly, medical professionals look for the traditional signs associated with the final stage of liver disease to diagnose alcoholic cirrhosis. It is likely that these patients will not accurately share their alcohol consumption, thereby making conversations with friends and family important in estimating the amount of alcohol typically consumed by the patient.

Portal hypertension complications, like hepatic encephalopathy, variceal bleeding, and ascites, can be present in patients with alcoholic cirrhosis. There are no clear findings in pathology that distinguish the advanced liver disease was caused by alcohol or from several other causes. This is especially true when the patient is in the final stage of alcoholic cirrhosis but does not have acute alcoholic hepatitis.

The combination of clinical acumen, laboratory values, and physical findings are an accurate method for clinically diagnosing alcoholic liver disease. A biopsy of the liver is not always necessary, but it can be acceptable in some cases. Typically, when it is uncertain if this is the correct diagnosis, a medical professional will require a biopsy. It is likely that more than 30% of patients are inaccurately clinically suspected of alcoholic hepatitis. Performing a biopsy can confirm the diagnosis. In addition, a biopsy can assist in making decisions on liver therapy, offer a prognosis, determine the amount of damage present, and also rule out additional unanticipated liver disease causes.

Non-Alcoholic Fatty Liver Disease or NAFLD

The non-alcoholic fatty liver disease has a few different forms and serves as a broad-based term for a range of liver conditions. Simple fatty liver disease indicates that the liver has high levels of stored up fat, but may not come with any damage to this liver or inflammation. The simple fatty liver usually will not get worse and doesn't cause any major health issues pertaining to the liver and is the most common type in people with NAFLD.

Non-alcoholic steatohepatitis, or commonly called NASH, is an additional type. NASH means the liver will have inflammation and possible damage to the liver cells. Both the inflammation and cell damage can lead to serious health problems such as liver cancer, cirrhosis, and scarring of the liver and liver failure. NASH is a much less common type of NAFLD but heavy use of alcohol causes damage that is comparable to the damage of NASH.

The common presence of non-alcoholic fatty liver disease is common in the Western nations, but it is spread throughout the globe. In fact, the non-alcoholic fatty liver disease is the most usual chronic liver disease in the U.S. today. It mainly affects people in their 40s and 50s who have type two diabetes or may be at a greater risk of heart disease. Metabolic syndrome, including increased belly fat, high blood pressure and triglycerides, and the body's ability to use insulin, are closely linked to the non-alcoholic fatty liver disease.

A non-alcoholic fatty liver disease may be symptomless at first, or forever. When symptoms of the disease are present, they can comprise liver enlargement, extreme feeling of tiredness or discomfort in the right side of the abdominal area near the liver.

Signs of non-alcoholic steatohepatitis and cirrhosis include large blood vessels beneath the skin, and swelling in the spleen or abdomen, skin, and eyes that begin to turn a yellow color, reddening of the palms and growth of breasts in men. With these symptoms present, making an appointment with a doctor is crucial.

It is unclear to experts why some patients develop a build-up of fat in the liver and others do not develop this illness. In addition, experts are unsure why some cases involve inflammation, which leads eventually to cirrhosis, and other cases do not. The following common links between non-alcoholic steatohepatitis and non-alcoholic fatty liver disease are:

1. Patients who are obese or overweight
2. Patients with a resistance to insulin. Resistance to insulin means your cells do not absorb sugar because of how it responds to the hormone called insulin.

3. Patients with hyperglycemia, or high blood sugar. Patients presenting with this symptom have type 2 diabetes or are pre-diabetic.
4. The patient's blood has high levels of triglycerides or increased fat levels.

A combination of these different issues a patient could present with can lead to the fat build up in the liver. Occasionally, some patients develop fibrosis, or their liver's scar tissues build up because their liver becomes inflamed and non-alcoholic steatohepatitis occurs. This happens when the patient's body reacts to the increased fat levels as a toxin.

Risk Factors

There are many conditions and illnesses that can raise your risk of developing the non-alcoholic fatty liver disease. Some of these risk factors include:

- Hypothyroidism or a thyroid that is underactive
- Hypopituitarism or a pituitary gland that is underactive
- Type 2 diabetes
- Sleep disorders such as sleep apnea
- Polycystic ovary syndrome
- Abdominal fat concentrations in obese patients
- Metabolic syndrome
- Elevated blood fat, especially triglycerides
- High cholesterol

People most at risk for developing non-alcoholic steatohepatitis include:

- The elderly
- Patients with diabetes including type 1 and type 2

- Abdominal fat concentration in a patient of any weight, however, it is more likely in overweight and obese patients.

Additional testing is necessary to tell the difference between non-alcoholic steatohepatitis and non-alcoholic fatty liver disease. The tests most often used include aspartate transaminase and elevated alanine transaminase. Additionally, many experts will use imaging studies to assist them in diagnosing a patient with non-alcoholic fatty liver disease. Ultrasonography and tomography are two of the more frequently used imaging types when diagnosing nonalcoholic fatty liver disease, however, neither of the procedures can distinguish steatosis and steatohepatitis.

Experts are in controversy over the use of a liver biopsy to diagnose non-alcoholic fatty liver disease. Medical professionals who argue that a liver biopsy is unnecessary cites the following reasons:

1. Risks associated with a biopsy.
2. Few conventional therapies that are available and effective.
3. The disease is generally benign.

There are few risks associated with conducting a liver biopsy, but as many as 30% of patients report transient pain, nearly 3% of patients report severe pain. Less than 3% of patients who undergo a liver biopsy experience substantial complications. Despite the controversy over conducting a routine biopsy, it is generally recommended that patients with advanced liver disease should get a biopsy.

In addition, patients that make significant lifestyle changes but still have continually elevated liver enzymes should be considered for a liver biopsy. The patient should be included in the decision to conduct a liver biopsy and it is recommended by the American Gastroenterological Association to base the decision to conduct a biopsy on each individual case and that the timing should be appropriate for the care of the patient.

Liver Cancer

Cirrhosis is the primary complication of both non-alcoholic steatohepatitis and non-alcoholic fatty liver disease. Cirrhosis is fibrosis or advanced-stage scarring, in the liver. Injury to your liver, like non-alcoholic steatohepatitis inflammation, causes the liver to respond in the form of cirrhosis. Fibrosis or scar tissue is developed by the liver to combat and lessen the inflammation it is experiencing. As inflammation persists, scar tissues continue to build in the liver. Cirrhosis that remains untreated can develop:

- Final-stage failure of the liver. This means that liver ceases all function.
- Liver cancer.
- Hepatic encephalopathy or speech becomes slurred and the patient becomes drowsy and confused.
- Esophageal varices or the veins in the esophagus become swollen. This can result in ruptured veins and internal bleeding.
- Ascites or abdominal fluid buildup.

Patients diagnosed with non-alcoholic steatohepatitis have a 20% chance of progression to cirrhosis.

In the United States, one of the primary causes of hepatocellular carcinoma is NAFLD or non-alcoholic fatty liver disease. Between 2004 and 2009, hepatocellular carcinoma in patients with fatty liver disease rose 5% every year. In addition, patients with fatty liver disease have shorter survival times than those without and when they are diagnosed, the tumor is often more advanced than those who develop this cancer without fatty liver disease. Because of the advanced complications of the fatty liver disease, hepatocellular carcinoma liver transplant is less common.

In a study conducted over a span of five years, liver cancer patients with fatty liver disease were often diagnosed at an older age, were typically Caucasian, and had advanced tumors. Their survival rate for fatty liver disease-related liver cancer was also four months less than those without the fatty liver disease. The study conducted on these patients is extremely significant due to the substantial amount of participants.

Cirrhosis is an indication of liver cancer, but not always, especially if the patient has the fatty liver disease. That is what makes it so challenging to detect and why the mortality rates are poor. A patient that has the fatty liver disease and is obese will typically be monitored more frequently than patients within a normal weight that have the fatty liver disease, primarily because the combination of the two diseases can be a higher risk.

Chapter 2: How the Liver Functions and Types of Liver Disease

Only vertebrae have a liver. No matter the vertebra that has a liver, its role is similar. Specific metabolites are detoxed from the body, proteins are synthesized, and digestion is aided by the production of biochemicals. In humans, it also is responsible for regulating the storage of glycogen, decomposing red blood cells, and producing various hormones.

Located over the intestines, right-hand kidney, and stomach and under the diaphragm is your liver. It takes up the right section of your abdomen's cavity. There are several functions this deep red-brown organ fulfills. Blood enters the liver from two primary avenues: the hepatic portal vein delivers blood rich in nutrients, and the hepatic artery delivers blood filled with oxygen.

The double lobes of the liver each have their own eight sections. Within each various section, there are about one thousand lobules. The common hepatic duct is made up of large ducts that splinter into smaller ducts with connected lobules on the ends. The function of the common hepatic duct is to move the liver cell's bile to the beginning portion of the small intestine called the duodenum, and the gallbladder. Hepatocytes are primarily contained in the liver's tissue. These regulate a large number of reactions of high-volume biochemical. These reactions include complex and small molecules being synthesized and broken down. Many of these reactions are paramount to the body's vital functions.

The liver expels the bile it produces, but the liver also monitors the blood and adjusts the chemical content as needed. Bile is critical in breaking down the fat in order for the body to be able to absorb and digest the necessary nutrients. The liver monitors all the blood that passes through from the intestines and stomach. When the blood enters the liver, the liver determines any imbalance and adjusts it as needed as well as passes on nutrients necessary to healthy bodily function.

Many medications are designed to be broken down and dispersed through the liver. The liver is effective at delivering the medication into the blood in the easiest way for the body to process it. The liver provides some of the most vital functions for the body. The following list contains a short list of the most recognizable functions of the liver:

1. Holds on to and disperses glucose when the body needs it.
2. Delivers fat to the body by producing unique proteins and cholesterol.
3. Develops specific proteins necessary for the plasma in blood.
4. Assists the digestive process beginning in the small intestine by breaking apart fats and removing waste due to the production of bile.
5. Holds on to iron to assist in processing hemoglobin.
6. Urea ammonia, which is harmful to your body, is converted into waste. Urine removes the end-product of the metabolism of protein, urea.
7. Cleanses the blood from harmful toxins like drugs.
8. Ensures that any blood clotting is regulated.
9. Eliminates bloodstream bacteria and develops immune factors to assist the body in resisting various infections.

10. Helps the body remove bilirubin stores. If the body holds on to too much bilirubin, the eyes and skin turn a yellowish hue.

The bloodstream or bile ferries harmful toxins out of your body after the liver has broken them down. Feces leave the body from the intestine, which is filled with the by-products of bile produced by the liver. If a by-product of the bile is filtered through the kidneys first, it leaves the body in the form of urine.

The liver is a gland that assists in digestions because if creates this bile. The bile created is what the body uses to break down fat and is an alkaline compound. When the fat is broken down, lipids remain. Bile emulsifies the lipids, which is how it helps digestion. For many years the function of the organ directly below the liver, the gallbladder, had an unknown necessary function. However, continued research shows that the gallbladder helps the liver by storing bile. No one is certain to this day how many functions the liver undertakes in a humans lifetime, but some texts estimate it has about 500 different roles.

If the liver ceases to function properly, there are a few options for treatment. Over the long term, it is unknown how it is best to make up for the loss of function in the liver. Short-term liver dialysis appears to be beneficial but it is not a long-term solution. There are no artificial livers that have been developed to replace or support a failing or failed liver. The only feasible long-term solution at this time for a failed liver is a liver transplant.

What Are the Different Types of Liver Disease?

The cause of the specific problem is what is used to classify the various types of liver disease. Hepatitis, or liver inflammation, leads to most of the various liver diseases. Hepatitis ranges from life-threatening and chronic to not serious and acute. Other times the issue is an associated part that impacts the function of the liver, for example, the bile duct. This means the disease or issue does not lie in the liver itself but can cause the liver to stop functioning correctly.

Viral Infections

Viral infections are one of the most typical developments of liver disease. These infections inflame the liver, and it is mainly due to hepatitis. Viral infections are classified as A, B, C, D, or E based on the various strains. Hepatitis B is a viral infection transmitted by blood or sexual contact. Hepatitis A is transmitted by food.

Parasitic Liver Infections

Over time the liver can also be damaged by parasites that infect the liver. Liver flukes or blood flukes, different types of flatworms or trematodes, are the most common parasitic liver infection. Snails, cattle, and sheep are the most common carriers for these worms. Humans contract these worms when they ingest food or water that has eggs or immature worms in it.

Alcoholic Liver Disease

Drinking alcohol over extended periods of time is another cause of liver disease. Excessive alcohol consumption leads to damage and inflammation of the liver. A patient with this disease typically has abused alcohol for a length of time and leads to liver failure. Sometimes this disease can be caught in its early stages and can be slowed down when alcohol consumption is stopped. Hepatitis from alcohol is toxic hepatitis.

Alcohol is not the only cause of toxic hepatitis. Several other chemicals can damage and inflame the liver. Some of these chemicals include over-the-counter and prescription drugs, herbal and nutritional supplements, and industrial chemicals like herbicides and cleaning supplies.

Autoimmune Repercussions

When your boy begins attacking itself, it is known as autoimmune hepatitis or autoimmune liver disease. Sometimes it is unknown as to why the immune system attacks the liver and the body, while other times it can be traced back to a source. For example, there are certain genes that can cause this to occur. After a prolonged attack by the immune system, the liver finally becomes inflamed and damaged. Primary sclerosing cholangitis and primary biliary cirrhosis are examples of autoimmune diseases that can cause this form of liver disease.

Genetic Disorders

Genes and genetic disorders are often inherited and lead to various forms of liver disease. Families often experience generational issues with their liver function. Some of these genetic liver diseases include Wilson's disease, hyperoxaluria, and hemochromatosis. Different substances build in the liver when a patient suffers from one of these types of diseases. Copper builds in the liver in patients with Wilson's disease, for example.

Growths, Tumors, and Cancer

The liver can also have a variety of growths and tumors as well as cancer. The growths can be both non-cancerous and benign or can be cancerous or malignant. Hepatocytes, the cells in the liver, cause a liver cancer called hepatocellular cancer. A benign tumor is sometimes a liver adenoma. Another benign tumor is a liver abscess. A liver abscess causes pus to build in the tissue of the liver. Cancer in the bile duct can prevent the liver from functioning properly, but it can also spread to the liver.

Cirrhosis

When the liver becomes scarred and the tissue is destroyed, it is called cirrhosis. This is the final stage of liver disease. Long periods of liver disease or alcoholic hepatitis are two of the most common reasons for cirrhosis to occur. When this occurs, it cannot be reversed. Cirrhosis will lead to death eventually.

Pediatric Liver Conditions

In infants and children, the liver can present symptoms but typically only if it is severely damaged. This is because the liver can regenerate and its reserve capacity is large, especially in children. Some of the liver diseases that are common in children include benign tumors, hepatic hemangioma, Langerhans-cell histiocytosis, alagille syndrome, progressive familial intrahepatic cholestasis, biliary atresia, and alpha-1 antitrypsin deficiency. Benign tumors are considered to be congenital and are the predominant form of liver tumors in children.

A polycystic liver disease is another disorder that begins at gestation and builds throughout the patient's life. It is a genetic disease, meaning, it runs in the family line. This disorder causes several cysts to appear in the tissue of the liver. These cysts typically appear later on in life. They are also typically asymptomatic. All these diseases, including those listed above, can lead to the derangement of the liver's process.

Signals of Liver Issues

The degree and symptoms experienced with liver disease vary from person to person and disease to disease. Despite this, the resulting action on the liver produces common signs even if there are no other symptoms. This is especially true when the disease is in an early stage.

Jaundice or Yellowed Eyes and Skin

One of the most common signals that there is something wrong with the liver is the discoloration of the eyes and skin. A patient suffering from a liver disease will often have a yellow tint in the whites of their eyes and throughout their skin. The yellowing skin color and eye discoloration are called jaundice. When the blood breaks down, red blood cells creates bilirubin that the body needs to excrete. This is usually removed through bile. When the liver is not functioning correctly, it does not excrete this thereby causing the discoloration because the bilirubin begins to build throughout the body. In addition to the yellow color, the skin may become itchy.

Dark Urine And/Or Pale Stool

In addition the yellowing of the skin and eyes, stool and urine may become discolored. Bile leaves the body usually through stool and some through urine, which is how bilirubin is normally excreted. The bilirubin and bile are why stool is a brown color. When the liver is not functioning and bilirubin is building in the body, it is not being excreted through the stool or urine. When this happens, stool color becomes paler. The kidneys begin compensating for the excess bilirubin and try to flush it out more through the urine. This makes the color of urine darker.

Pain in the Liver

The intensity and nature of pain in the liver can vary, and it does not occur in every liver disease. Pain in the liver is located below the right ribcage, in the top right-hand side of the abdomen. Most people's livers sit in this location in their body. A small part of the liver does extend over the middle of the body into the left upper part of the abdomen, so it is possible to also feel pain here, but it is uncommon.

Easy to Bruise

Another signal that there is something wrong with the liver is being able to bruise easily. This symptom can be related to a variety of issues, so it is not isolated directly with liver disease; however, it can indicate something is wrong with the liver. This is especially likely if easy bruising happens alongside any of the other symptoms listed above. Blood clotting is controlled in part by the liver when it is functioning properly. When it is not, the liver could potentially be unable to create enough proteins to clot the blood and prevent bruising. This is why bruising can occur easily, even if the injury was the only minor.

Additional Signals to Watch out For:
- Extreme tiredness or fatigue.
- Abdomen swelling with excess fluid or ascites.
- Additional swelling with excess fluid not in the abdomen.
- No or little appetite.
- Episodes of vomiting or nausea.

Liver Disease Diagnosis

Tests are typically run on a patient when liver disease is suspected. These tests typically include blood tests. These tests look for specific markers. For instance, inflammation or injury appears in the response of the liver by the production of acute-phase reactants.

Chapter 3: What Is a Liver Detox?

Before you embark on a liver detox, it is important that you are aware of the variety of forms a detox can take and also the associated precautions. Liver flushes cleanse or detoxes, terms typically used interchangeably, are a method of supporting your liver remove toxins. Some programs even claim it can purge gallstones!

Prior to beginning any liver detox program, make sure to review what symptoms could occur, what signs you need to be aware of that could indicate an adverse reaction, and what could lead to potentially harmful situations.

There are many detoxes or flushes you can choose from and this variety opens the door for some plans to be labeled as safe and effective when in reality it is harmful and ineffective. Be aware of what choices are available and use your best judgment before beginning any new dietary or lifestyle plan.

The Most Common Liver Detoxes

1. Master Cleanse, AKA the Lemonade Diet
   A diet focused on minor starvation, participants only drink a special lemon drink for ten days while supplementing with laxatives and salt water to assist in defecation. Starvation diets are popular for a variety of reasons but unfortunately, they do worse things for your body than good. They slow down your metabolism and can cause other health concerns like dehydration and disrupted microorganisms. Using laxatives can lower

electrolytes and interfere with bowel movements. Laxatives can also interrupt the normal microorganism activity, disrupting digestive functions. Another potentially deadly side effect of this diet, especially when used repeatedly, is elevated acid in the blood, called metabolic acidosis. This diet can disrupt the balance of alkaline and acid in the body, causing severe health complications. Another complication is the production of gallstones. Finally, the overuse of laxatives can create damage to the gastrointestinal tract and develop a dependency on laxatives for elimination.

2. Colon Irrigation, AKA Colonic
Like an enema, this flush involves flowing water through a tube that is inserted in the rectum to flush out the colon. The purpose is to help remove toxin build up in the colon. The problems with this type of flush are the uncomfortable side effects. For example, vomiting, nausea, bloating, and cramping are all reported, even when an experienced professional do the procedure. Dehydration is another common side effect. More serious health concerns include perforated bowel, colon or bowel infections, and dangerously altered electrolyte levels.

3. Gallbladder or Liver Flush
Randolph Stone is credited with this detox. Stone instructed his participants to mainly eat apples and drink apple juice. They were to only eat fruits and vegetables and drink herbal tea and olive oil. In addition, they were supposed to inject a laxative, typically water with Epsom salt. This form of a detox is dangerous because it is a form of fasting and also overuses laxatives. Both practices can be very dangerous to your health. In addition, targeting

the liver in such a way can potentially release a gallstone from the gallbladder. For people who have gallstones, many are unaware of them until they become lodged in the duct of the gallbladder. When this occurs, it is very painful and emergency surgery is required.

4. Eat Liver-Cleansing Food, AKA the Detox Diet
   Some foods are loaded with additional toxins that can "bog down" the liver. For example, foods like sugar, chemicals, fat, and alcohol, can all burden the liver. On this diet, these types of foods should be avoided. Instead, participants focus on foods that support the liver, like apples, walnuts, artichoke, dandelion, grapefruit, and lemon. This is a safe approach to detox, especially when it is paired with an appropriate intake of calories, carbohydrates, and protein.

5. Herbal Supplements for Detox
   Many nutraceuticals are available to assist in liver detox. For example, turmeric, vitamin C, N-acetyl-cysteine, alpha R-lipoic acid, and milk thistle have all been shown to support the liver. At the cellular level, the various supplements assist with the detox. In addition, they can protect against damage. It is possible to have a sensitivity or allergy to the various herbal supplements. Before taking anything new, make sure to read and adhere to the instructions. Also, be aware of any reaction or adverse effect it may cause.

Common Detox Symptoms

In addition to the symptoms outlined above, the following symptoms are common while engaging in a liver detox:

- Influenza or the common cold

- Congestion in the sinus cavity
- Trouble sleeping
- Aching body
- Bad-smelling feces
- Diarrhea
- Cough
- Mental fog or confusion
- Irritable
- Anxious
- Dizzy spells
- Acne
- Skin reactions
- Intense or different body odor
- Extreme tiredness or fatigue

Most of the time, these symptoms are an indication that your body is removing toxins from the fat cells throughout the bloodstream. If the symptoms are not severe, they will normally subside once the body has removed all the toxins.

It is typical for some people to react differently to cleansing than other people. Prior to starting a liver detox, make sure to consult your healthcare professional. Seek a physician's support and guidance, especially if you have one or more of the following conditions:

- Chronic liver or kidney disease.
- Problems with the colon, including colon cancer, Crohn's disease, diverticulitis, or Irritable Bowel Syndrome.
- Seniors or children.
- Breastfeeding or pregnant women.
- Cardiac disease.
- Hypoglycemia.
- Diabetes.

The Best Detox Solution for You

The most beneficial detox, flush, or cleanse that you could do to support and heal your liver is to eat the best foods and rink the best beverages to aid and ease your liver. This means having a focus on nutritional foods including adequate amounts of water. It is important to avoid fasting or starvation diets including the use of laxatives. These are not beneficial to your body including your liver. If you choose to include an herbal supplement, make sure you choose a reputable brand and source to help protect and support your liver.

It is not simple to detox the liver, and sometimes it is not a pleasant process. But the outcome can be crucial to your longevity and overall health. Despite the many options available for a liver detox, there are some that are not as safe as others. Prior to dedicating yourself to a strict regime, make sure you look into the plan thoroughly and keep an eye out for any negative side effects you are experiencing. This is especially important if you suffer from a chronic illness. If you suffer from something like this, make sure you also work closely with your healthcare providers so you can participate in a gentle and healthy method that is best and most effective for you.

Chapter 4: The Benefits of a Liver Detox

It is common to disregard liver detoxes, but there are several benefits attached to this practice. It spurs healthy eating and also helps you lose unwanted or unneeded weight. Below are some of the most common benefits of a liver detox:

1. Lose unwanted and unneeded weight.

    Fat is broken down in the digestive system by bile, which is produced in the liver. If weight loss is your goal, starting with a liver detox could be a good starting point because this process promotes the production of bile.

2. Support the immune system.

    To have a strong immune system, your liver needs to be healthy. This is because one of the many roles of the liver is to lower toxins in your body. A liver detox can result in boosting your immune system.

3. The risk of liver stones is minimized.

    Excessive levels of cholesterol in the diet can lead to the development of liver stones. Bile hardens when there is excess cholesterol and this hardened bile turns into small stones. These small stones can then restrict the function of the gallbladder and liver. In some cases, you can have as many as 300 liver stones preventing your liver's function! During a liver detox, it is possible and likely to remove 100 to 300 liver stones from your body.

4. A whole body detox is supported.

Toxins always exist at some level in your liver because of its role in the body's function. It is designed to eliminate toxins by converting them into a byproduct that is harmless to your body. A healthy level of toxins is normal and typically does not create a problem in your body. The problems begin to occur when the toxins build up. To make sure your liver is functioning the way it should, you need to detox your liver.

5. Energy is increased.

After the liver breaks down toxins into a harmless byproduct, some of the byproducts are used in the body as a nutrient. However, if the liver is blocked with problems like liver stones or toxin build up, these key nutrients never make it to your blood. When your blood does not get the nutrients it needs, you can experience fatigue. To help increase your energy, detox your liver. In addition to experiencing the boost in energy, you will also know that your body is getting the nutrients it was missing before.

6. Vitality improves.

To return to your ideal proficiency, a liver detox is necessary. Your skin will appear healthier and brighter when you reduce your toxins that have built up in your liver. Your body will respond better to exercise when you support bile production. Some patients and participants feel and appear to be five years younger when they complete a liver detox!

Chapter 5: How to Detox Your Liver Through Diet

The accessibility of fast food, which is often unhealthy and quick, makes any diet or lifestyle change difficult. In order to make changes in your diet, you need to restrain yourself and hold yourself accountable. If you can do this, you can experience life-changing benefits in many areas of your overall health. To detox your liver through diet, consider the following tips:

Tip 1: Eliminate or Minimize Foods That Are Toxic to Your Body

Some foods work against your liver health such as processed foods when your diet includes many of these foods frequently. Processed foods contain ingredients like refined sugar and hydrogenated oils. Foods like processed lunchmeats and convenience foods are known for their toxicity and harmful effects on your body. Hydrogenated oils, or trans fats, contain increased levels of saturated fat. The oil's chemical structure has been engineered to improve the life of the product it is added to. A diet rich in trans fats increases the likelihood of cardiac disease by over 25%. Additionally, it is theorized that trans fats lead to inflammation in the body because it interferes with your immune system.

Other serious health conditions are linked to foods like lunchmeats, fast foods, and convenience foods, which commonly contain added nitrites and nitrates. The purpose of these additives is to retain color in the foods, prohibit the growth of bacteria, and increase the shelf life of the product. Instead of consuming these types of foods, you need to replace them with healthier options that support your liver function. It sometimes requires a little creativity to make healthier options to mimic and replace these unhealthy foods, but you can develop meals that you and your family find full of flavor and supports your liver.

For example, instead of purchasing processed lunchmeats, slice your own roasted turkey or chicken. Homemade granola bars, mixed nuts, carrot sticks, celery sticks, and fresh fruit are all good options to replace a bag or a handful of chips. Instead of making a box of mac and cheese, find a recipe for a healthy alternative such as cheesy spaghetti squash. Potassium, pantothenic acid, manganese, B vitamins, and niacin are all present in spaghetti squash. In addition, spaghetti squash is low in saturated fat and calories. You can add a garnish of crushed walnuts on top to provide a punch of antioxidants and omega-3 fatty acids to also support your heart health.

When you eat foods that are processed, in addition to changing your diet, you also need to ensure that your digestive enzymes properly function. When your liver enzymes are not balanced, you can develop liver and digestion illnesses like Crohn's disease.

Tip #2: Juice Made from Raw Vegetables Is an Effective Delivery Method of Nutrients

A liver detox requires a large number of raw vegetables in your diet, but increasing to the required servings can be impossible for some people. To assist you in getting the vegetable servings you need in an easy way is to juice raw vegetables. One glass of fresh, raw vegetable juice can deliver as much as five servings of raw vegetables that you need. In addition, if you do not like eating raw vegetables, juice can be a tastier and easier way to get the nutrients you require.

Another benefit of raw vegetable juice is that it is easier for your liver to digest. It also makes the nutrients in the vegetables easier for your body to absorb. Some of the most beneficial vegetables in liver detox include Brussels sprouts, cauliflower, and cabbage. The flavors of these vegetables may not sound appetizing; however, you can include other raw vegetables to alter the flavor. Vegetables that are good to add for additional nutrients and flavor include leafy greens, beets, cucumbers, and carrots. All these vegetables assist in developing a balanced pH level by lowering the levels of acid in the body.

Finding a flavor combination you prefer will take some experimentation. Consider adding other fresh, raw juices or fresh herbs to develop a unique flavor. Some flavorful herbs include mint and parsley. One of the most beneficial raw vegetable juices to your liver detox is from organic carrots. Beta-carotene, a nutrient that converts to Vitamin A, is found in carrots. Vitamin A is essential for flushing toxins out of your body as well as reduces liver fat. Ginger root is another beneficial additive to raw vegetable juice. Ginger supports digestion and is anti-inflammatory. Oranges also add a great, sweet and/or tangy flavor to juice. Additionally, oranges deliver Vitamin B6, Vitamin A, and Vitamin C.

Vegetable juice contains a large amount of fiber. High amounts of fiber support your digestion and speed up your elimination process. Having speedy elimination of toxins means your body does not have time to store these, which can build up and harm you.

Tip #3: Foods Rich in Potassium Are Essential

You need to eat over 4,500 milligrams of potassium every day. Are you positive you are getting this recommendation consistently? Probably not! Foods that contain higher levels of potassium help you lower your cholesterol, support your heart's health, supports your liver cleanse, and reduces your systolic blood pressure. There are potassium supplements available, but you should try to obtain your potassium recommendation through healthy foods such as sweet potatoes, tomato sauces, greens, beans, bananas, and molasses.

Sweet Potato

Many people immediately think that they need to eat more bananas to increase their potassium intake; however, sweet potatoes are actually the richest source of potassium. In addition to beta-carotene and a high amount of fiber, one medium-sized sweet potato delivers about 700 milligrams of potassium. Sweet potatoes are also low-calorie but contain high levels of iron, magnesium, and the vitamins B6, C, and D. Sweet potatoes also have a naturally sweet flavor from natural sugars. The natural sugars are dispersed slowly through the bloodstream thanks to the function of the liver. The beauty of this natural process is that it regulates itself, preventing blood sugar spikes that refined sugars cause.

Tomato Sauce

Tomatoes also contain several nutrients including potassium. When tomatoes are delivered as a paste, puree, or sauce, the benefits of tomatoes are more significantly concentrated. For instance, a cup of fresh tomatoes offers about 400 milligrams of potassium, but a cup of pureed tomatoes contains over 1,000 milligrams! To make sure you get the most benefits in a paste, puree, or sauce, select organic tomato products.

If you intend to make your own concentrate, consider the following recipe to get the most from your effort and the fruit's nutrients:

Ingredients:

- Organic tomatoes, halved

Directions:

1. Warm your oven to 425 degrees Fahrenheit. Place the halved tomatoes on a baking sheet face down.
2. Roast the tomatoes until the skin begins to shrivel.
3. Remove the pan from the oven and allow the tomatoes to cool.
4. Once cool, pinch or slide off the skins and place flesh into a blender or food processor. Pulse tomatoes to gently crush.
5. Pour the crushed, roasted tomatoes into a sieve or strainer to remove seeds, if you prefer. Strain as often you prefer or need.
6. Pour the strained mixture into a Dutch oven or large stock pot on your stovetop. Simmer the sauce for up to 2 hours or until the sauce is thick. Remember, the sauce will continue to thicken after you remove it from the heat, so cease simmering just before the sauce reaches the consistency you prefer.

Leafy Greens

One cup of spinach or beet greens contains a large number of antioxidants and more than 1,300 milligrams of potassium. These ingredients are easy to add to raw juice and can powerfully support the liver. To add these to your diet, chop the vegetables and add to your juice mixture or sprinkle on top of salads. You can also sauté quickly on your stovetop. Additionally, beet greens help the flow of your bile and cleanse the gallbladder naturally.

Beans

There are multiple healthy beans you can choose from to add to your diet. Beans contain a large amount of potassium in addition to fiber and protein. Beans like lima beans, kidney beans, and white beans are all great options and good alternatives to other beans, such as garbanzo beans. Instead of making hummus from garbanzo beans, try one of the other beans in your recipe and enjoy your new creation with celery sticks and carrot sticks.

Molasses

Just any molasses is not the best source of potassium; however, blackstrap molasses can provide a significant portion of your recommended daily value of potassium in addition to other nutrients like copper, manganese, calcium, and iron. In fact, just 2 teaspoons of blackstrap molasses provide about ten percent of the recommended amount of potassium.

An easy way to incorporate blackstrap molasses into your diet is by replacing other sweeteners you use. Use it in porridge made with quinoa, on top of steel-cut oatmeal, or make homemade BBQ sauce with it. Even stirring the two teaspoons into your morning coffee is an excellent way to add sweetness as well as nutrients. The added benefit of adding blackstrap molasses to your coffee is that it enriches the flavor while reducing the acidic taste.

Banana

Bananas are rich in potassium. Adding a single medium banana to a smoothie is a great way to increase your potassium and sweeten the drink. A medium banana delivers about 470 milligrams of potassium, digestion support, and release of heavy metals and toxins from your body. When you are going through your liver detox, these benefits are essential. Make sure you always have enough bananas on hand to add to your foods or to snack on during your detox.

Tip #4: Do an Enema with Coffee

An enema assists with constipation, but an enema with coffee also helps you regain more energy and support your liver detox. Enemas target the bottom part of the large intestine. There are many ways and resources to help you complete it at home, unlike other interventions, like a colonic. Colonics target the full bowel and requires the assistance of a professional. This makes an enema a more accessible and "attractive" action to assist in your liver detox. You can purchase an enema kit at most drug or convenience stores.

When doing a coffee enema, organic coffee is kept in your bowel. By retaining it in your lower part of the large intestine, it allows the wall of the intestine to absorb the coffee liquid and transport it to the liver. The absorption of the organic coffee stimulates the production and flow of bile. This stimulation kick starts your liver and gallbladder. When your liver and gallbladder are kick-started, you begin to produce glutathione, a chemical compound that is a strong cleaner. This chemical compound aids in the elimination of the toxic build up in your body.

Moving out toxins quickly is essential during your liver detox. To give yourself a coffee enema, boil three cups of distilled or filtered water with 2 tablespoons of ground, organic coffee. Once the mixture reaches a boil, lower the heat and simmer for about 15 minutes. When done, let the mixture cool to room temperature. Once the coffee mixture is completely cool, strain it through a cheesecloth to remove all the sediment from the liquid. Use this liquid in your enema kit. Once the liquid is inserted, aim to keep the liquid in for up to 15 minutes. When you reach 15 minutes or your limit, release.

Tip #5: Supplements for Turmeric, Dandelion, and Milk Thistle Are Beneficial

Turmeric

Various health conditions, such as chronic pain, prostate health, breast health, osteoarthritis, depression, cancer, and Alzheimer's disease, are all subjects of current scientific research being conducted on the effect of turmeric on these conditions. Preliminary results already show that turmeric can support liver metabolism and tissue, regulates the balance of our blood sugar, assists digestions, minimizes pain in the joints, and helps minimize depression. More benefits are expected to emerge as research is continually published.

Dandelion

Many people who have to maintain any sort of lawn hates dandelions. This weed moves freely and infests the ground every spring and throughout the summer. While it may be a nuisance in the yard, these little flowers contain beneficial minerals and vitamins from its pedals to its roots. When you ingest dandelion, you help your liver detox easier by acting as a diuretic and speeding up toxin elimination. Additionally, dandelion helps upset digestion, heartburn, unbalanced blood sugar levels, and a weakened immune system. You can take dandelion root as a supplement or drink it in an herbal tea for your liver detox.

Milk Thistle

An ideal detox herb is milk thistle. Many familiar with this herb consider it the "king" of herbs used for detox. This is why it is so important and valuable during your liver detox. Part of the benefit of consuming milk thistle includes removal of alcohol in the liver, pollutants from the environment, prescription medicines, and heavy metal build up. For patients undergoing radiation or chemotherapy, they experience a series of unwelcome side effects, which milk thistle can help reduce. To support the regeneration of the liver, the silymarin active in milk thistle is beneficial to the strength of the liver's cellular walls. Take a milk thistle supplement or drink it in an herbal tea designed for your liver detox.

Bonus! Burdock Root

Similar to dandelion, this root is helpful with detoxing your blood, which then aids the function of the liver. Similar to milk thistle, burdock root can also be taken as a supplement or in a liver detox tea.

Tip #6: Take Liver Supplements or Eat Organic Liver Meat Regularly

Consuming organic liver meat from young and healthy chicken or cattle that is grass-fed contains the most coQ10, chromium, zinc, copper, iron, choline, and folic acid, vitamin A, and B vitamins. The get the most nutrients from a food, you cannot do better than eating liver.

If eating liver is not an option, ingest beef liver supplements. Make sure to choose supplements that offer a guarantee that no antibiotics, pesticides, or hormones are used in the care and feed of the animals. This ensures you get the best and most nutrients in the supplements.

Chapter 6: Natural Remedies for Fatty Liver Disease

Currently, there are only two primary therapies offered for NAFLD. The first is using medications and pharmaceutical interventions. The second is intervening in your lifestyle. Intervention includes engaging in or increasing physical exercise, modifying your diet, or reducing your body weight. The most common therapy is lifestyle intervention, specific modifications to your diet and reducing your body weight. These two often go hand-in-hand. Metabolic diseases, such as hyperlipidemia and obesity, as well as NAFLD, can be slowed through moderate and long-term exercise.

Despite the knowledge that intervention in your lifestyle can reduce the progression of NAFLD, the mechanisms underlying this benefit are still unknown. Several published scientific studies illustrate the benefits of lifestyle intervention, but none firmly put a finger on the reason for it. Still, it is undeniable the potential for therapeutic benefits. These natural interventions, or remedies, have more beneficial outcomes in scientific studies than pharmaceutical interventions. Pharmaceutical therapy includes various drugs, including renin-angiotensin system blockers, lipid-lowering agents, insulin sensitizers, and antioxidants. Some studies on animals and cells show promising results, but few clinical trials on humans are positive.

There are several beneficial effects in herbal remedies for NAFLD cessation. Attention to these natural remedies has increased in recent years because they are available around the world; typically have little or no side effects, and multiple clinical and basic studies support their effectiveness.

Current Natural Remedy Findings for Treating NAFLD

Goji Berry, Wolfberry, or Lycii Fructus

From the Solanaceae family, goji berry is the fruit from the Lycium Barbarum. Chinese medicine made this fruit famous for its benefits on the eyes and liver. The LBP, or the polysaccharide part of the fruit, is the most beneficial part of the goji berry. Results of modern studies show that LBP has a variety of benefits biologically, including a reduction in the risk tumors, maintenance of glucose metabolism, neuroprotection, immunoregulation, and antioxidant abilities.

Additional clinical studies show that the juice of LBP increases the amount of immunoglobulin G, levels of interleukin-2, and lymphocytes in humans. Reducing the formation of lipid peroxide and increasing antioxidant serum levels are additional benefits of LBP.

Early findings show that LBP prevented propagation and encouraged hepatoma cells apoptosis in the liver. An additional study illustrated LBP's protective attributes when incorporated in a diet high in fat that caused oxidative stress injury in the liver. In these situations, LBP increased the activity of antioxidant enzymes and the products of oxidative stress to help protect against further oxidative stress injury in the body. Other studies showed the powerful healing properties of LBP in alcohol-related fatty liver disease and how it can aid in the regeneration of the liver.

Garlic or Allium Sativum

There is a long history of medicinal and culinary uses of garlic in the Mediterranean region, Egypt, and Asia. A recent report published that eating a whole piece of garlic helped improve blood glucose resistance, lipid metabolism, and oxidative stress. Reduced activity of the cytochrome P450 system and increased antioxidant activity resulted in one study when black, aged garlic was combined with the administration of chronic ethanol in rats. Garlic has also been found to help protect and repair liver damage from CCl4. When paired with other medicinal and natural remedies, garlic enhances the beneficial effects of reducing steatosis, inflammation, oxidative stress, and fibrosis. Finally, garlic also helps prevent further damage to the liver for patients with NAFLD.

Green Tea

Another natural remedy is the green tea plant. This remedy is one of the most documented plants used to prevent liver problems. In the last two decades, increased attention on the beneficial and healing properties of this plant has supported its capabilities in liver health. The plant Camellia Sinensis provides the leaves used in making green tea. The plant was originally found in China but it spread across Asia to places like Vietnam, Korea, and Japan. It has now spread to Western locations, infiltrating into black-tea cultures.

Mice treated with CCl4 were also given pure EGCG, or epigallocatechin-3-gallate, in one impactful study. EGCG is green tea's primary polyphenol. The result showed benefits on a biochemical and histological level. It impacted inflammation, oxidative stress, and helped resolve liver injury. In another recent study, EGCG was shown to prevent the entrance and passage of hepatitis C. Obese lab rats in a study conducted on liver disease and EGCG found benefits on both the health of the liver and the reduction of unwanted weight.

Resveratrol

Red grapes contain a phytoalexin that can be extracted, which is called resveratrol. It is well documented to protect against inflammation and oxidative stress. It is one of the most accepted natural remedies because of its powerful properties and its worldwide availability. Recent studies have shown that resveratrol is an effective treatment for NAFLD. This is an effective remedy to use every day to prevent and heal fatty liver disease.

Milk Thistle

As mentioned in the previous chapter, milk thistle is a beneficial plant during a liver detox. Milk thistle is in the daisy family and produces two important derivatives, silymarin, and silybin. There have been more than 10,000 reports published over the past ten years on the benefits of milk thistle on the body, and specifically liver health. The findings in these reports link the effects of the two derivatives to hepatoprotective, chemopreventive, and antioxidant results. In the liver specifically, silymarin and silybin improve the effects of antioxidants. They also, directly and indirectly, impact fibrosis and inflammation in the liver. An additional study shows that patients suffering from chronic hepatitis C and NAFLD, they experienced better effects of silymarin because of the increased concentrations of flavonolignan plasma and wide-ranging enterohepatic circulation.

Additional Decoctions and Derivatives to Consider

Additional natural remedies that have been used in traditional Chinese medicine and are now supported through experimental biology, pharmacology, and chemistry, include berberine. The herb Coptidis Rhizoma from China contains this isolated alkaloid, which has an anti-steatotic effect. It also reduces the inflammation response from hepatitis. Currently, there are no modern studies directly linking berberine to the treatment of NAFLD.

Additional Natural Suggestions

- Minimize sugar intake to less than 30 grams per day.
- Reduce stress.
- Slow down your pace of living.
- Place a castor oil pack over the liver a few times a week.
- A couple times a week eat organic organ meats.
- First thing in the morning drinks eight ounces of beet kvass.
- Incorporate low-impact and stress-relieving physical activity such as yoga or walking into your weekly activity.

Chapter 7: Healthy Diet Foods and Drinks for Fatty Liver Disease

Almost one-third of the adult American population is affected by fatty liver disease. It is on the primary causes of liver failure and once the liver fails, there is no long-term treatment option other than a liver transplant. Many cases of the fatty liver disease are not diagnosed until late in the disease, making some of the damage irreversible. However, it is possible to prevent and treat the disease to improve your length and quality of life. One of the most common methods of prevention and treatment includes dietary changes. It does not matter if you have an alcoholic fatty liver disease or non-alcoholic fatty liver disease, diet can improve your liver's health.

The general rules to follow for a liver-healthy diet includes:

- Do not consume alcohol.
- Consume a very small amount of saturated fats, refined carbs, trans fats, salt, and sugar.
- Modify your diet to include several whole grains and plants that are high in fiber, such as legumes.
- Eat large amounts of vegetables and fruits.

Because the fatty liver disease is a build-up of fat in the liver, reducing the additional fat you intake is important. You can also focus on reducing your caloric intake to aid in weight loss, which can also help relieve fatty liver disease and additional stress on your body. When you lose unwanted weight, you lower the risk of contracting the fatty liver disease. If you are overweight, set the goal to lose about 10% of your current body weight.

How to Heal Fatty Liver Disease Through Food

Listed below are some of the best foods and drinks you should consume during a liver detox and while supporting your healthy liver function.

1. **Coffee**

   You are welcome, coffee lovers! Reports have shown that drinking coffee helps reduce unusual enzymes in the liver. In addition, patients with fatty liver disease that also drink coffee regularly often have less damage to their liver than those that do not drink it. Moderate amounts of caffeine can minimize abnormal liver enzymes, which is especially important for people who are at risk of developing the fatty liver disease.

2. **Leafy greens**

   These superfoods also block the buildup of fat. For example, broccoli prevented fat build up in the liver in rats in one study. Spinach, kale, and Brussels sprouts also aid in weight loss. Look for recipes that use a lot of leafy greens to get a powerful punch every day.

3. **Tofu**

   Tofu is a good source of protein and is also low fat, but it is the soy protein in the food that specifically benefits those suffering from fatty liver disease. Rats in a study at the University of Illinois revealed the power of tofu and soy protein in protecting against the fat build up in the liver.

4. Fish

Lower inflammation and improve the fat levels in the liver with the support of omega-3 fatty acids. These beneficial acids can be found in foods like trout, tuna, sardines, and salmon. These are all considered "fatty" fish but they provide a healthy fat that your body can break down easily versus other fats that are easily stored in the liver. When preparing fish, remember to focus on keeping the recipe low-fat because the fish already contain enough fat for your body.

5. Oatmeal

When you are struggling with fatigue as a side effect of fatty liver disease or during the early stages of treatment for the disease, it can be hard to function properly. Eating whole grain carbohydrates like oatmeal can provide your body with a boost of energy that can sustain for long periods of time. In addition, the fibers in oatmeal help make you feel full and sustain that feeling of fullness. Finally, oatmeal has also been shown to assist you in maintaining a healthy body weight.

6. Walnuts

Another food high in omega 3s is walnuts. When patients with fatty liver disease consume a small handful of walnuts, often they have better liver test results.

7. Avocado

Protect your liver by eating healthy fats like those in avocados. Current research shows that avocados contain specific chemicals that potentially reduce damage to the liver. Avocadoes are also a rich fiber source, which also aids in losing weight.

8. **Low-fat dairy and milk**

   A study published in 2011 on rats reported that whey protein in milk can help protect against liver damage, even if damage already exists. Consume a glass of milk per day or about eight ounces of organic, grass-fed animal cheese for optimal results.

9. **Sunflower seeds**

   Vitamin E is high in sunflower seeds and is known for its antioxidant properties. Antioxidants help your liver protect itself from further damage.

10. **Olive oil**

    A third source of omega 3s on this list. Choose this oil instead of butter, shortening, or margarine while cooking. Olive oil has also been shown to control healthy weight levels and reduce the level of liver enzymes.

11. **Garlic**

    As mentioned earlier in this book, garlic is helpful in protecting and supporting the liver as well as promoting healthy body weight. It is also very flavorful so it can make many dishes delicious quickly. It is a good source for burning built up and unwanted fat in the body.

12. **Green tea**

    Another repeat food on our list, green tea has been shown to help you absorb and process fats in the body, rather than storing them in your liver. It has also been linked with improved liver function. Other benefits include sleep assistance and reduced cholesterol.

Additional Liver-Supporting Foods

- Beets
  Rich in antioxidants and activates liver enzymes, also improves bile production and improves physical activity.
- Organic apples
  Rich in fiber, especially with the skin on, and make sure the fruit is organic because apples tend to be one of the top fruits and vegetables to have excessive amounts of pesticides on them.
- Broccoli sprouts
  Strong detoxifier, rich in antioxidants, boosts glutathione more than just broccoli, contains a hormone regulator called indole-3-carbinol, and contains cancer-fighter sulforaphane.
- Fermented foods such as sauerkraut, kefir, kombucha, kimchi, or pickles. Promotes digestion and elimination through good bacteria compounds.
- Citrus fruits such as lemons, limes, oranges, or grapefruit. Helps the liver cleanse and create enzymes for detox.
- Carrots
  Rich in beta-carotene and plant-flavonoids, and contain Vitamin A for liver disease prevention.
- Most forms of vegetables.
  Cauliflower and broccoli contain glucosinolate for detoxing enzyme production and sulfur for overall health in the liver. Spinach and other leafy greens are rich sources of chlorophyll to assist in removing toxins from the blood and also provide an alkaline balance to the heavy metals in the liver.

Additional Liver-Supporting Beverages

- Blueberry juice: Fibrosis, which is the scarring that is the result of liver disease, was the topic of the study published in the journal PLOS One on March 2013. The animals in the study were fed blueberry juice to observe the effects it has on fibrosis over a period of eight weeks. The results of the study indicate that blueberry juice has the ability to both increases the liver's capacity to stand levels of oxidative stress and increase proteins that support the liver to fight against fibrosis. Oxidative stress occurs when cells are damaged by free radicals which are unstable molecules.

- Blood orange juice: In 2012, a study published in the World Journal of Gastroenterology concluded that fat accumulation is prevented when participants regularly consumed blood orange juice. Over the span of 12 weeks, the obese animals in the study were fed the juice every day. According to the study, the rats experienced several healthy responses, including improved insulin sensitivity, reduced triglycerides, and overall cholesterol, lowered body weight, as well as provide protection against fat build up in the liver. The hormone, insulin, regulates blood sugar levels. It is important that the body is sensitive to this hormone so it can regulate blood sugar appropriately. If the body does not have a stable sensitivity to the insulin, it is possible and likely the person will develop diabetes.

- Noni fruit juice: Noni is a plant that grows in tropical climates and bears noni fruit. It is botanically known as Morinda Citrifolia. Health stores are the primary vendors for noni juice supplements in the United States. It is likely that you will find noni juice mixed with other fruit juices, most commonly grape juice. The conclusion from the

2008 study on animals that was published in the journal Plant Foods and Human Nutrition shows damage from toxins in the liver is minimized when the participants drank noni juice regularly.

- A note on fruit juice: Fruit juices often contain added refined sugar. Make sure to read the labels carefully. Choose juices that have no or little sugar added and also look for the juice content. Try to purchase juices that are labeled as 100% juice, if possible. Many juice brands will include only a small portion of fruit juice in their bottle. This often occurs with blueberry juice. Juice also contains high caloric levels and the fiber from the fruit has been removed. You will get far less fiber than if you were to eat the whole fruit by itself. For those interested in juicing your fruit, keep in mind that some fruit is only available seasonally. For example, blood oranges are in stores from the month of January through the middle of April. If you can find them in stores outside of those times, they will most likely be more expensive and not great quality.

Avoid the Following Foods:

1. Salt: Too much salt makes your body retain water. Make sure not to consume more than 1,500 milligrams per day.
2. Red meat: These culprits are sources of unwanted saturated fats. Beef and deli meats specifically should be avoided.
3. White pasta, rice, and bread: White foods indicate that it has been processed. Processed foods raise your blood sugar and lack fiber and other nutrients that their whole grain counterparts offer.
4. Fried foods: Anything fried will be high in calories and unhealthy fats.
5. Additional sugar: Fruit juices, sodas, cookies, and candy are all high in refined and added sugar. These raise your blood sugar and can increase fat build up in your liver.

An Example Diet Plan

The next chapter will cover meal plans and recipes in more depth, but provided below is a sample meal plan to illustrate what a fatty liver diet and detox can look like.

Meal Time	Breakfast	Lunch	Dinner	Snacks
Menu	8 ounces of coffee with skim or low-fat milk 1 cup of whole-grain oatmeal topped with 2 tablespoons almond butter and 1 medium banana, sliced	8 ounces low-fat milk 1 medium apple 8 ounces steamed broccoli, carrot, or other leafy green 1 small baked potato 3 ounces grilled chicken 1 cup fresh spinach topped with olive oil and balsamic vinegar	8 ounces steamed broccoli, carrots, or another vegetable 8 ounces mixed fresh berries 8 ounces of low-fat milk 1 whole-grain roll 3 ounces of baked salmon a small mixed-bean salad	2 teaspoons of hummus with fresh vegetable sticks 1 tablespoon almond butter spread over sliced fresh apples

Additional Natural Remedies Suggestions for Fatty Liver Disease

Other natural remedies to consider do not include diet. These changes can improve your overall health, including your liver function. Some of these remedies include:

- Increasing your physical activity.
  When you pair a diet with exercise, you not only lose the excess and unwanted weight, but you also can manage your general health and liver disease with this combination. The goal should be a minimum of 30 minutes of moderate to high-activity several days a week.
- Reduce your cholesterol.
  If you are not able to lower your cholesterol through diet and exercise alone, you may need to work with your healthcare professional to begin certain medications to assist you. It is important to lower your triglyceride and cholesterol levels. You can do this through your diet by minimizing or eliminating added sugar and saturated fats.
- Keep diabetes in check.
  The fatty liver disease often accompanies diabetes and vice versa. Changing your diet and your physical activity levels are effective treatment methods for these two diseases. If these two remedies do not drop your blood sugar levels to a healthy level, you should speak with your healthcare professional to stabilize your blood sugar with medication as well.

Chapter 8: Eating Plans and What Foods and Drinks to Avoid

Have you decided that this is the weekend you are doing a liver detox or cleansing? If you are still on the fence about the idea, maybe you should put it on your agenda. A detox has the reputation of being a life-disrupting and challenging undertaking, but a short detox focused on healthy foods is easier and less painful than you are probably imagining. Your liver is an incredibly important organ in your body, and your skin is the only larger organ you have. A detox is a way you can help it function better every day by giving it a break from foods that are hard to process, that are filled with preservatives and are toxic to your health. Your liver supports most of your bodily functions including your digestion, reproduction, immunity, and hormones. Even your skin is supported by your liver function.

It can do all of this work because of the nutrition it derives from what you eat. Juice diets are a common detox method used to help your body remove toxins, but they are challenging to stick to. Dietitians and nutritionists are now more likely to suggest and support a food-based cleanse. A detox that focuses on foods that provide your liver with the "right" nutrients makes it easier for participants to stick to, especially if they are new to detoxing. It is far easier and less of a commitment than doing a traditional juice cleanse. In addition, during a juice cleanse, participants often struggle with metabolic slowdown and withdrawal and deprivation feelings. Doing a food-based detox; however, minimizes these side effects.

Foods to Avoid in Your Liver Detox Eating Plan

The great news is that you can eat during your detox! You get to eat a lot of great foods and counting calories is not really the focus of the plan. Instead, you are focused on increasing the "good" while minimizing or eliminating the "bad." Below is a list of the few types of foods you need to avoid while participating in your cleansing:

1. Soy products, except for tempeh if you typically consume soy products.
2. Corn
3. Red meats or other fatty meats. If you eat meat regularly stick to lean, roasted chicken breast.
4. Canola and vegetable oils.
5. Coffee
6. Alcohol
7. Condiments like ketchup and mayonnaise.
8. Foods high in sodium or added salt.
9. Processed or fried foods.
10. Gluten products like pasta and bread.
11. All dairy products.
12. Foods high in sugar especially added refined sugar. Fruit and its natural sugar are ok in moderation during the detox.

Tips on How to Get the Most from Your Liver Detox Eating Plan

Before you whip up recipes and plan out your weekend of meals, consider the eight tips below before you get started so you can get the most out of your time.

1. Plan on drinking eight ounces of water with a fresh lemon wedge the first thing in the morning. This helps get your body hydrated and ready to flush out the stagnant toxins from overnight.

2. Drink half your body weight in water every day. Consider adding a teaspoon of chlorophyll or spirulina powder to eight ounces of water to boost your detox. You can add this to your water up to three times a day during your detox.

3. Choose organic foods whenever you can to help cut out added hormones and toxins.

4. Sprinkle flax or chia seeds on your foods. These contain a rich dose of fiber, which helps your colon remove the toxic waste from your liver. You can also create a flax tea by steeping 1 tablespoon of flax in eight ounces of hot water, then straining the liquid to remove the seeds before drinking.

5. Stock up on foods that are liver-healthy such as cilantro, parsley, watercress, spinach, cucumber, radish, broccoli, asparagus, lime, lemon, and apple. These can be easily eaten on the go or added to other foods for additional flavor and benefits.

6. Plan to make a green smoothie or juice every day. The liquid state helps your body digest the nutrients and also allows your liver to absorb what it needs for optimal health. Consider adding a cup of spinach or leafy greens to a handful of other fruits and vegetables for a lunch alternative or afternoon "snack."

7. Two hours before bedtime, you should stop eating. Your liver works through the night to remove toxins from your body while you sleep so do not give it an overload right before it starts its hardest work.

8. Allow yourself to get all the rest you need. Sleep helps your body reset and restore, so make sure you give it the time while you detox. When you focus on resting, your body can promote the ideal function of all your organs, including your liver, and support your digestion.

Eating Plan Menu and Detox Plan Sample

Friday Evening

Begin by going to the grocery store and purchasing the fresh foods you need for this weekend. Eat a filling, healthy dinner with a lot of vegetables and about three ounces of a lean protein, preferably fish like salmon or tuna. Before you go to bed, prepare a chia seed pudding with a handful of fresh fruit on top for an easy morning meal tomorrow. As you settle into bed, drink eight ounces of filtered water with a fresh lemon wedge or a cup of turmeric tea. Make sure you go to bed early enough so you can get eight hours of good sleep.

Saturday Early Morning

First thing, when you wake up, drink eight ounces of filtered water with a fresh lemon wedge or a cup of unsweetened green tea. Eat your chia seed pudding, and add seeds or nuts to the top, if you prefer. Walnuts, pistachios, sunflower seeds, or pumpkin seeds are all good options. These nuts or seeds will help add fiber to the meal and also help you stay fuller for longer.

Saturday Late Morning

If you are beginning to feel hungry but it is too early for lunch, prepare a green smoothie or fresh green juice. Make sure to include a leafy green with fruits and vegetables with no added sweetener. Bananas and unsweetened coconut milk are good options to add a little sweetness naturally.

Saturday Afternoon

For lunch, cook kelp noodles and top with sliced vegetables in a rainbow of colors. Consider orange and purple carrots, beets, bell peppers, etc. If you need protein and more filling foods, roast the tempeh to add in the top of the salad. On the side, slice an organic apple with a dollop of unsweetened almond butter for dipping.

Saturday Late Afternoon

If you begin to feel hungry after lunch but it is too early for dinner, grab a handful of carrot stick or another fresh vegetable. A small handful of walnuts, cashews, or almonds are another good afternoon snack. Sip on lemon water throughout the day, especially if you are feeling hungry but you have just eaten something. Your body is most likely thirsty, not hungry if this is what you are feeling after a meal or snack.

Saturday Night

Prepare a healthy meal full of vegetables and seeds. Consider adding fresh vegetables to a large butter lettuce leaf spread with unsweetened almond butter and sprinkled on top with sunflower seeds. Enjoy a glass of organic or homemade kombucha. Before going to bed, place a castor oil pack over your liver and then treat yourself to a warm Epsom salt bath. Head to bed at a good time to make sure you get your full eight hours of sleep.

Sunday Early Morning

Pour yourself a bowl of gluten and grain-free muesli mixed with unsweetened almond or coconut milk. Top it with fresh fruit and seeds, if you prefer. Sip on a cup of green tea or mix fresh blueberries, a lemon wedge, and cucumber slices into eight to ten ounces of filtered water to drink.

Sunday Afternoon

Spiral cut a zucchini to make a "zoodles" and toss with a fresh pesto made with herbs, olive oil, crushed walnuts, and garlic. Serve with a bowl of cool avocado soup.

Sunday Late Afternoon

For a snack, enjoy a sliced apple or radish or prepare a homemade hummus with liver-healthy beans and serve it with sliced vegetables. Fill your afternoon with light activity such as meditation or yoga or a short, leisurely walk. Make sure to drink plenty of filtered water flavored with lemon or cucumber.

Sunday Night

Top a large, leafy green salad with 1/3 cup tempeh, roasted chicken, or beans and a balsamic vinegar and olive oil dressing. In your blender, add one cup of spinach with blueberries, pineapple, and a banana to make a tasty green smoothie to drink. Before bed, place another castor oil pack over your liver and take another Epsom salt bath, if you would like. Make sure you go to bed at a decent time so you can get your full eight hours of sleep again.

Monday Morning Through Night

Continue a modified detox breakfast so you do not shock your body with old, unhealthy foods. Instead, enjoy ½ avocado sliced on top of scrambled eggs or another chia seed pudding with nuts, seeds, and fresh fruit. Drink eight ounces of water with a lemon wedge or a cup of green tea before any coffee. Try to continue eating many fruits and vegetables throughout the day and do not drink any alcohol tonight.

A 24-Hour Liver Detox

If you are not interested or able to do a weekend detox, consider doing a 24-hour cleanse. The week leading up to the day of your cleansing, make sure you eat a lot of the following foods:

- Celery
- Beets
- Asparagus
- Citrus fruit
- Brussels sprouts
- Broccoli
- Cauliflower
- Lettuce
- Cabbage
- Kale

Avoid alcohol and processed foods leading up to the day of your cleanse as well. On the day of your cleansing, make 72 ounces of the following liquid to drink throughout the day. Also, make sure to drink at least 72 ounces of water.

24-Hour Detox Drink

Ingredients:

- Cranberry juice
- Nutmeg
- Ginger root
- Cinnamon
- Fresh orange juice from 3 oranges
- 3 Lemons

Directions:

1. In a large container, mix three parts water to one part cranberry juice.
2. In a large saucepan, steep ¼ teaspoon grated ginger root, ¼ teaspoon nutmeg, and ½ teaspoon cinnamon in four cups of water. Simmer for 20 minutes.
3. Let cinnamon, ginger and nutmeg liquid cool to room temperature.
4. Juice the oranges and lemons into the liquid and stir to combine.
5. Combine the infused liquid with the cranberry juice and stir well.

Easy Detox Soup Recipes

Broccoli Soup

Ingredients:

- Coconut oil, 1 Tsp.
- Broccoli florets, 2 cups
- Celery stalks, chopped, 2
- Parsnip, peeled and chopped, 1
- Garlic cloves, minced, 2
- Carrot, peeled and chopped, 1
- Onion, chopped, 1
- Low sodium vegetable stock, 2 cups
- Spinach, 2 cups
- Lemon, juiced, ½
- Chia seeds, 1 tbsp.
- Sea salt, ½ tsp.
- Mixed nuts and seeds, toasted, if preferred.

Instructions:

1. In a large stockpot, warm the oil over low heat. Combine the broccoli, celery, parsnips, carrots, garlic, and onion and cook for five minutes. Stir often.
2. Pour in the broth and boil. Cover with a lid and lower to a simmer. Simmer for 7 minutes or until vegetables are cooked but not too soft.
3. Mix in the spinach and then pour mixture into a blender. Add the lemon and chia seeds. Blend until creamy.
4. Add salt as preferred and serve with warm, toasted nuts and seeds, if desired.

Beet Soup

Ingredients:
- Beets, medium, cubed, 3
- Coconut oil, 1 Tsp.
- Carrots, diced, 2
- Leek, small, diced, 1
- Garlic cloves, minced, 1
- Onion, diced, 1
- Vegetable stock, warm, 2 cups
- Sea salt, ¼ tsp.
- Chia, pumpkin, and sunflower seeds, if preferred.

Instructions:

1. In a large stockpot, place the beets inside and cover with water. Bring to a boil and then lower the heat. Simmer uncovered for 30 minutes or until the beets are tender.
2. Drain the beets from the water and allow it to cool.

3. In a large skillet, warm the oil over low heat. Combine the carrot, leek, garlic, and onions and cook for seven minutes. Place vegetables on a plate to cool.
4. In the blender, combine the beets, vegetables and warm stock. Blend until smooth.
5. Add salt as preferred and serve with warm, toasted nuts and seeds, if desired.

Conclusion

Thank you for making it through to the end of *Fatty Liver Diet – Guide on How to End Fatty Liver Disease*, let's hope it was informative and able to provide you with all of the tools you need to achieve your goals whatever they may be.

The next step in preventing or healing fatty liver disease is to break out your calendar and decide when you are going to start your liver-healthy diet. If you are unsure about how you will do with making a life-changing diet, start with the 24-hour detox. Pick up a few of the ingredients and choose a day to focus on your liver. If you feel ready for more of a challenge, block out a weekend for the 2½ day diet. Whatever you decide, just make sure you decide to focus on improving your liver function and heal fatty liver disease.

After you figure out when you are going to do your detox, continue to stay focused on your liver health. Continue to boost your health by nourishing your body through healthy meals. Review the liver-supporting foods listed throughout this book and stock your fridge and pantry with things you can integrate and grab when you need to. Make it easier on yourself to always have these foods on hand and a few recipes you can rely on when you are in a pinch. Give the recipes in the last chapter a try, but come up with a few of your own based on your own food preferences.

The diet plan in the last chapter is designed to give you quick and easy options to help you cure fatty liver disease and support your liver healthy. The liver detoxes here are focused on providing your body with the nutrients it needs as well as support the liver's health. As you have learned, this is not a book about how to lose weight while doing an unhealthy (and inefficient) liver detox. This is about supporting your health and liver by curing fatty liver disease. If you struggle with fatty liver disease or another liver issue, it is important that you make the suggested changes to your diet, not just when you are completing a liver detox, but as often as possible. Follow your fatty liver diet and enjoy the benefits of a healthier, happier you.

BONUS:

As a way of saying thank you for purchasing my book, please use your link below to claim your 3 FREE Cookbooks on Health, Fitness & Dieting Instantly

https://bit.ly/2LEQVu2

You can also share your link with your friends and families whom you think that can benefit from the cookbooks or you can forward them the link as a gift!

Printed in Great Britain
by Amazon

36054284R00043